TRENDS IN SOUTHEAST ASIA

The **ISEAS – Yusof Ishak Institute** (formerly Institute of Southeast Asian Studies) is an autonomous organization established in 1968. It is a regional centre dedicated to the study of socio-political, security, and economic trends and developments in Southeast Asia and its wider geostrategic and economic environment. The Institute's research programmes are grouped under Regional Economic Studies (RES), Regional Strategic and Political Studies (RSPS), and Regional Social and Cultural Studies (RSCS). The Institute is also home to the ASEAN Studies Centre (ASC), the Singapore APEC Study Centre and the Temasek History Research Centre (THRC).

ISEAS Publishing, an established academic press, has issued more than 2,000 books and journals. It is the largest scholarly publisher of research about Southeast Asia from within the region. ISEAS Publishing works with many other academic and trade publishers and distributors to disseminate important research and analyses from and about Southeast Asia to the rest of the world.

"BUILDING A SAILBOAT IN A STORM"

The Evolution of COVAX in 2021 and Its Impact on Supplies to Southeast Asia's Six Lower-Income Economies

Khairulanwar Zaini

ISSUE

4

2022

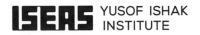

YUSOF ISHAK
INSTITUTE

Published by: ISEAS Publishing
                  30 Heng Mui Keng Terrace
                  Singapore 119614
                  publish@iseas.edu.sg
                  http://bookshop.iseas.edu.sg

ISEAS Library Cataloguing-in-Publication Data

Name(s): Khairulanwar Zaini, author.
Title: "Building a sailboat in a storm": the evolution of COVAX in 2021 and its impact on supplies to Southeast Asia's six lower-income economies / by Khairulanwar Zaini.
Description: Singapore : ISEAS-Yusof Ishak Institute, February 2022. | Series: Trends in Southeast Asia, ISSN 0219-3213 ; TRS4/22 | Includes bibliographical references.
Identifiers: ISBN 9789815011418 (soft cover) | ISBN 9789815011425 (pdf)
Subjects: LCSH: COVID-19 (Disease)—Vaccination—International cooperation. | Drug accessibility—Southeast Asia. |
Classification: LCC DS501 I59T no. 4(2022)

Typeset by Superskill Graphics Pte Ltd
Printed in Singapore by Mainland Press Pte Ltd

FOREWORD

The economic, political, strategic and cultural dynamism in Southeast Asia has gained added relevance in recent years with the spectacular rise of giant economies in East and South Asia. This has drawn greater attention to the region and to the enhanced role it now plays in international relations and global economics.

The sustained effort made by Southeast Asian nations since 1967 towards a peaceful and gradual integration of their economies has had indubitable success, and perhaps as a consequence of this, most of these countries are undergoing deep political and social changes domestically and are constructing innovative solutions to meet new international challenges. Big Power tensions continue to be played out in the neighbourhood despite the tradition of neutrality exercised by the Association of Southeast Asian Nations (ASEAN).

The **Trends in Southeast Asia** series acts as a platform for serious analyses by selected authors who are experts in their fields. It is aimed at encouraging policymakers and scholars to contemplate the diversity and dynamism of this exciting region.

THE EDITORS

Series Chairman:
　Choi Shing Kwok

Series Editor:
　Ooi Kee Beng

Editorial Committee:
　Daljit Singh
　Francis E. Hutchinson
　Norshahril Saat

"Building a Sailboat in a Storm": The Evolution of COVAX in 2021 and Its Impact on Supplies to Southeast Asia's Six Lower-Income Economies

By Khairulanwar Zaini

EXECUTIVE SUMMARY

- In the first half of 2021, COVID-19 vaccine doses from the COVAX Facility were in short supply, and the plan to mass produce COVAX vaccines through the Serum Institute of India (SII) faltered as the pandemic surged in India in March 2021.
- Due to COVAX's shift in approach towards convincing richer nations to redistribute their excess doses, the second half of 2021 saw increases in the frequency and volume of its shipments. Donors were however able to "earmark" their dose donations and identify their intended recipients.
- The six Southeast Asian countries which qualified for free COVAX shots—Cambodia, Indonesia, Laos, the Philippines, Timor-Leste and Vietnam (the AMC6)—received 16 million doses in the first half of 2021. In the second half, they received 128 million doses from COVAX, 80.9 per cent of which were earmarked donations.
- Despite making up 7 per cent of the world population, the AMC6 collectively accounted for 24.3 per cent of all earmarked dose donations (and 25 per cent of the United States' total dose donations) to COVAX in 2021.
- The AMC6 greatly benefitted from COVAX's pivot to dose donations. This demonstrated the region's strategic salience to Washington and its allies, but came at the expense of vaccine equity, which the region has prudential reasons to care about.

- The execution of COVAX hammers home the hard truth that multilateral governance is a difficult act to pull off even with the best intentions and is not impervious to the geopolitical interests and agendas of the major powers.

"Building a Sailboat in a Storm": The Evolution of COVAX in 2021 and Its Impact on Supplies to Southeast Asia's Six Lower-Income Economies

By Khairulanwar Zaini[1]

INTRODUCTION

As it became increasingly evident that vaccines would be central to the recovery from the global pandemic, the COVID-19 Vaccines Global Access (COVAX) Facility was created to ensure equitable access to COVID-19 vaccines, especially for poorer countries. However, the erratic and delayed COVAX shipments in the first half of 2021 led to doubts about the Facility's ability to fulfil its pledge of securing and delivering 2 billion doses by the end of the year. In June, the Malaysian vaccine minister Khairy Jamaluddin derided it as an "abysmal failure".[2] Remarkably, by September 2021, the Facility was confident enough to forecast the allocation of 1.4 billion doses by the end of the year—with 1.2 billion of those to be disbursed gratis to lower-income countries.[3] COVAX's improved fortunes in the latter part of 2021 can primarily be

---

[1] Khairulanwar Zaini is Research Officer at the ISEAS – Yusof Ishak Institute, Singapore.

[2] Syed Jamal Zahiid, "Minister Khairy Tells World Bank to Speak Out Against Vaccine Inequity, Calls Covax 'Massive Failure'", *Malay Mail*, 23 June 2021, https://www.malaymail.com/news/malaysia/2021/06/23/minister-khairy-tells-world-bank-to-speak-out-against-vaccine-inequity-call/1984309

[3] "COVAX Global Supply Forecast", Gavi, 14 December 2021, https://www.gavi.org/sites/default/files/covid/covax/COVAX-Supply-Forecast.pdf

attributed to a surge in dose donations from wealthier countries, as they began releasing their excess inventory of vaccines.

This article will examine how the COVAX Facility evolved in 2021 over two distinct phases and the implications for six lower-income Southeast Asian countries.[4] In the first phase, which coincided with the first half of 2021 (1H), the COVAX Facility had to rely on its own ability to purchase vaccines from the manufacturers. In the second phase, from July onwards (2H), the Facility was instead sustained by dose donations from the West.

In the first phase, the supply of COVAX shots was scarce for Cambodia, Indonesia, Laos, the Philippines, Timor-Leste and Vietnam—the six Southeast Asian countries which qualified for free COVAX shots (hereafter referred to as the AMC6).[5] In 1H 2021, the AMC6 were promised 25 million COVAX doses, but the Facility only delivered 16 million doses, or 65.3 per cent of the AMC6's entitlement. The shift to the second phase significantly boosted the frequency and volume of COVAX shipments to the AMC6. In 2H 2021,[6] a total of around 128 million COVAX doses were shipped to the AMC6, with around 104 million (80.9 per cent) of these shots sourced from dose donations from wealthier countries.

However, as this paper will elaborate at the end, the Facility's evolution into its second phase (COVAX 2.0) does not entirely align with the goal of developing a truly multilateral institution to advance vaccine equity. Even though the AMC6 have handsomely benefitted

---

[4] The analysis is based on information sourced from public databases up to 15 December 2021, including the UNICEF COVID-19 Vaccine Market Dashboard (https://www.unicef.org/supply/covid-19-vaccine-market-dashboard).

[5] The "AMC6" designation reflects the coverage of the six countries under the COVAX Advance Market Commitment (AMC), the mechanism which provides free COVID-19 shots to lower-income economies. While Myanmar is also an eligible AMC recipient, it has been excluded from the foregoing analysis. This is because the COVAX Facility has not registered any shipment to the country (owing to the post-coup domestic political turbulence).

[6] The 2H and full-year figures in this article are up to 15 December 2021.

from COVAX 2.0, these immediate gains come with some future risks which should be acknowledged.

HOW THE "BEAUTIFUL IDEA" OF COVAX FALTERED

COVAX is the vaccines pillar of the Access to COVID-19 Tools Accelerator (ACT-A), an initiative launched in April 2020 to enhance collaboration between governments, global health organizations, the private sector, and other key stakeholders in addressing the pandemic. In tandem with its two other pillars (diagnostics and therapeutics), ACT-A is meant to shepherd and co-ordinate efforts to develop and produce COVID-19 tests, treatments and vaccines, and more importantly, to ensure equitable access to these medical resources globally.[7]

Under the stewardship of Gavi (formerly known as the Global Alliance for Vaccines and Immunization), the Coalition for Epidemic Preparedness Innovation (CEPI), and the World Health Organization (WHO),[8] COVAX's initial target was to deliver at least 2 billion doses

---

[7] The ACT-A is not a decision-making body or a new organization, but instead functions as a framework for coordination. Responsibility for the ACT-A is shared across eight co-convening agencies, which includes the World Health Organization (WHO), Gavi, the Coalition for Epidemic Preparedness Innovation (CEPI), and the World Bank Group. ACT-A also has a fourth pillar which focuses on strengthening healthcare systems against the pandemic. For a brief summary of the ACT-A, see "The ACT Accelerator: Heading in the Right Direction?", *Lancet* 397, no. 10283 (April 2021): 1419.

[8] The three co-leads each head the COVAX Facility's three "workstreams". CEPI is responsible for identifying the prospective vaccine candidates for the Facility to invest in, while Gavi is charged with procurement and delivery. The WHO (in particular, its Strategic Advisory Group of Experts on Immunization) oversees policy and allocation-related matters. The UNICEF is also involved in COVAX as a key delivery partner, given its long-standing experience in global vaccine procurement and distribution. For more details of COVAX's "loosely organized but institutionally complex" structure, see Katerini Tagmatarchi Storeng, Antoine de Bengy Puyvallée, and Felix Stein, "COVAX and the Rise of the 'Super Public Private Partnership' for Global Health", *Global Public Health* (2021): 5–7; https://doi.org/10.1080/17441692.2021.1987502

in 2021, with 950 million doses to be distributed gratis to lower-income countries and a further 100 million doses reserved as a "humanitarian buffer".[9] Central to this "beautiful idea" is the COVAX Facility, which would function as a "global procurement mechanism" and a "global vaccine hub".[10] The underlying concept is for the Facility to pool global resources and financial muscle in order to accelerate vaccine research and development, and to incentivize production and negotiate better deals with vaccine suppliers by capitalising on the Facility's significant economies of scale and collective purchasing power. The Facility would invest in a portfolio of promising vaccine candidates, assume responsibility for the global procurement of those vaccines, and then serve as a clearing house to allocate the doses equitably across the world. The plan was for the Facility to first provide all participating countries with sufficient doses to vaccinate 20 per cent of their populations.[11] Once all the countries have received their entitlements, the Facility would proceed to the next stage during which doses will be prioritized for countries still severely affected by the pandemic.

---

[9] The humanitarian buffer refers to the stock of vaccines kept for marginalized populations (such as asylum seekers and refugees) who find themselves in "instances of state failure and conflict". The remaining 950 million out of the 2 billion doses would be distributed to wealthier countries that have joined the COVAX Facility as "self-financing" participants. These figures were mentioned by Dr Seth Berkley, the chief executive of Gavi, in an online webinar in November 2021. See "COVAX Past, Present, and Future: A Conversation with Dr Seth Berkley", 15 November 2021, Centre for Strategic and International Studies (CSIS), Washington, DC, webinar, https://csis-website-prod.s3.amazonaws.com/s3fs-public/event/211117_Bliss_Berkley_COVAX_0.pdf?Rm9.P6HfquS2dzjmVZozoHq1fR7Bgiql

[10] Ann Danaiya Usher, "A Beautiful Idea: How COVAX Has Fallen Short", *Lancet* 397, no. 10292 (June 2021): 2322, 2325.

[11] According to the COVAX Facility, the first tranche of doses should go towards providing vaccine coverage to frontline healthcare workers and the vulnerable (such as the elderly), so as "to maximize the public health impact of such limited supplies". See "WHO Concept for Fair Access and Equitable Allocation of COVID-19 Health Products", WHO, 9 September 2020, p. 10, https://www.who.int/publications/m/item/fair-allocation-mechanism-for-covid-19-vaccines-through-the-covax-facility. More details about COVAX's allocation mechanisms, policies and principles can be found at https://www.who.int/groups/iavg

The Facility is designed to be sustained through two separate and distinct funding streams. The first involves higher-income countries buying their COVAX doses as "self-financing participants" (SFPs) and providing advance payments for their purchase options or commitments.[12] Brunei, Malaysia and Singapore are among the seventy-six countries that are part of this self-financing tier.[13] The Facility's second funding stream is the Advance Market Commitment (AMC), which would be sustained by donor grants, whose channels include official development assistance and private philanthropy. The AMC would secure the vaccines for ninety-two low and lower-middle income countries.

As of early November 2021, the AMC had raised around US$10.1 billion in donor pledges—enough for 1.8 billion doses—though not necessarily as cash in hand.[14] (Moreover, the timing of the donations

---

[12] Self-financing participants of the COVAX Facility can either undertake a "Committed Purchase Arrangement" to buy a specific number of doses or an "Optional Purchase Arrangement", which allows the participant to decline doses of a particular vaccine brand without sacrificing their full entitlement. Committed Purchases come with a lower upfront payment of around US$1.60 per dose (around 15 per cent of the cost). In contrast, Optional Purchases require an advance payment of US$3.10, along with a risk-sharing surcharge of US$0.40, for each dose. See "COVAX Explained", Gavi, https://www.gavi.org/vaccineswork/covax-explained (accessed 1 December 2021).

[13] Thailand had initially declined to participate in the COVAX Facility, since it did not qualify as an AMC recipient and was doubtful about the costs and reliability of COVAX supplies. In July 2021, however, Bangkok expressed their belated interest in entering COVAX as an SFP, but the country is not expected to receive any shots before 2022. See "Nakorn Says Not Joining Covax Wasn't a Mistake", *Bangkok Post*, 24 July 2021, https://www.bangkokpost.com/thailand/general/2153843/nakorn-says-not-joining-covax-wasnt-a-mistake; and Chalida Ekvittayavechnukul, "Thailand to Join COVAX, Acknowledging Low Vaccine Supply", *Diplomat*, 22 July 2021, https://thediplomat.com/2021/07/thailand-to-join-covax-acknowledging-low-vaccine-supply/

[14] As of April 2021, the AMC had been able to secure around US$7.4 billion in assured funding. The bulk of the post-April 2021 donation pledges came during the Gavi COVAX AMC Summit on 2 June, which raised an additional US$2.4 billion. See "World Leaders Unite to Commit to Global Equitable Access for COVID-19 Vaccines", Gavi, 2 June 2021, https://www.gavi.org/news/media-room/world-leaders-unite-commit-global-equitable-access-covid-19-vaccines

matter: the slow pace of funding commitments in 2020 prevented COVAX from exercising its procurement capacity until it was almost too late—an issue which will be discussed shortly.)

With its pledge of US$3.5 billion, the United States is the largest AMC donor, while Germany and Japan have committed around US$1 billion each (Figure 1). Singapore has donated US$5 million to the AMC, and despite being AMC-eligible countries themselves, the Philippines and Vietnam have respectively committed US$1.1 million and US$500,000 to the AMC as well.[15]

Importantly, vaccine purchases made by the COVAX Facility's self-financing participants would not "cross-subsidize" the procurement of doses for the AMC recipients—the latter is meant to be entirely donor-financed.[16] Thus, the Facility needs wealthier countries to not only donate generously to the AMC, but to also make a significant portion of their vaccine orders through COVAX, so that the Facility can obtain the purchasing power and scale to enjoy bulk discounts.

As Ann Danaiya Usher explains, the hope was that higher-income countries would "buy into COVAX as insurance", even if they pursued their own bilateral deals.[17] Usher further describes how Gavi had to tweak the arrangements to persuade rich countries to participate: self-participating countries were granted the option of choosing which particular vaccine they wanted to purchase from COVAX (instead of, as initially agreed, to be "product agnostic"), and the permission to purchase additional vaccines to cover up to 50 per cent of their populations

---

[15] These figures are correct as of 9 November and derived from "Key Outcomes One World Protected – COVAX AMC Summit", Gavi, https://www.gavi.org/sites/default/files/covid/covax/COVAX-AMC-Donors-Table.pdf (accessed 1 December 2021).

[16] "The Gavi COVAX AMC Explained", Gavi, https://www.gavi.org/vaccineswork/gavi-covax-amc-explained (accessed 1 December 2021).

[17] Usher, "A Beautiful Idea", p. 2322. Even Gavi's chief executive "actively promoted COVAX as a fallback option for those who had struck bilateral deals", as reported by Storeng, Puyvallée and Stein, "COVAX and the Rise of the 'Super Public Private Partnership'", p. 8.

Figure 1: Donors to the COVAX AMC

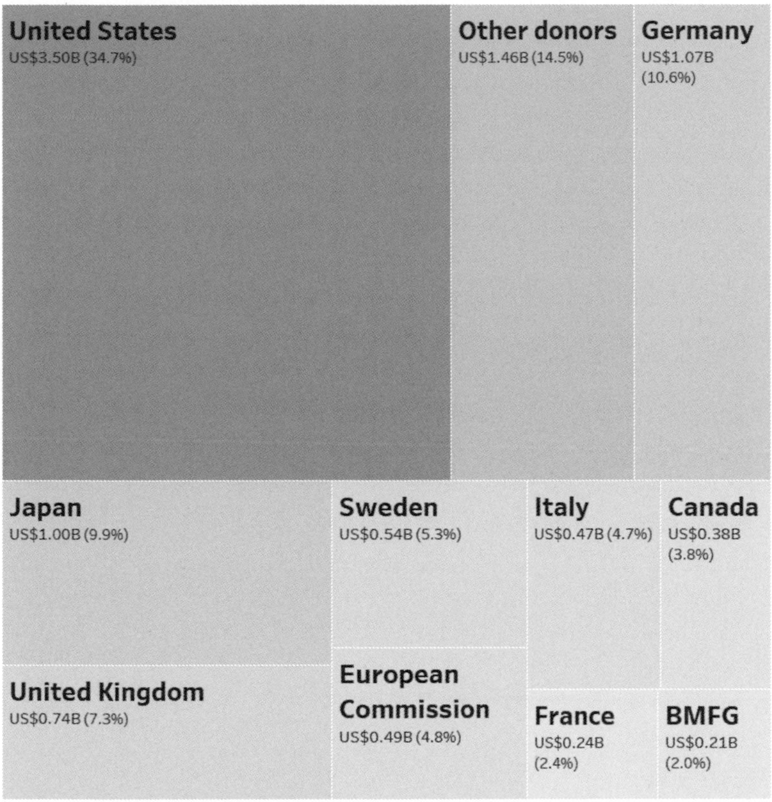

United States US$3.50B (34.7%)		Other donors US$1.46B (14.5%)	Germany US$1.07B (10.6%)
Japan US$1.00B (9.9%)	**Sweden** US$0.54B (5.3%)	**Italy** US$0.47B (4.7%)	**Canada** US$0.38B (3.8%)
United Kingdom US$0.74B (7.3%)	**European Commission** US$0.49B (4.8%)	**France** US$0.24B (2.4%)	**BMFG** US$0.21B (2.0%)

Note: BMFG is the Bill and Melinda Gates Foundation.

(a privilege not afforded to the AMC recipients, whose entitlements are still limited by the 20 per cent ceiling).[18]

The time taken to accommodate the demands of these rich countries, as well as the lack of "sufficient and readily available early funding",

---

[18] Usher, "A Beautiful Idea", p. 2323. A caveat is that even if the SFPs purchased COVAX supplies in excess of 20 per cent of their population, these countries would not be able to receive this excess supply until all the AMC recipients had received their 20 per cent entitlements.

meant that the COVAX Facility could not secure early access to the vaccines.[19] Dr Seth Berkley, Gavi's chief executive, revealed that it took "from June until December [2020] to raise the first $2.4 billion. And then to [the] middle [of] the next year [i.e., 2021] to raise the $10 billion that was necessary for the first tranche of doses".[20]

Meanwhile, wealthier countries concluded their own advance-purchase agreements with vaccine manufacturers to obtain supplies, leveraging on their ability to pay more than the COVAX Facility could afford.[21] The Facility did not stand a chance—global vaccine production capacity was almost fully reserved by the global North "even before COVAX secured its first financial instalments and was fit to start negotiations".[22] In particular, COVAX could only secure delayed access to a limited number of the newer mRNA vaccines. Moderna was apparently unavailable, and while the Facility did manage to order 40 million Pfizer/ BioNTech doses for 2021, only 1.2 million was promised for the first half of the year.[23]

Gavi was still able to kick-start COVAX by commissioning the Serum Institute of India (SII), its long-time partner and the world's largest vaccine manufacturer, to produce 1.1 billion doses.[24] On 24 February 2021, Ghana received the world's first COVAX shipment of 600,000

---

[19] Ibid.

[20] "COVAX Past, Present, and Future".

[21] Although self-financing participants form one of the two financial legs that COVAX stands on, their involvement later became a source of concern when the Facility faced supply constraints. For instance, Canada and Australia chose to exercise their COVAX purchase options despite already having secured vaccines through their bilateral deals. This kind of "double-dipping" leaves even fewer doses for the AMC recipients, which are more heavily dependent on COVAX.

[22] Storeng, Puyvallée and Stein, "COVAX and the Rise of the 'Super Public Private Partnership'", p. 7.

[23] "COVAX Past, Present, and Future".

[24] The SII had obtained the licence to produce the AstraZeneca vaccine locally, under the brand name of Covishield.

AstraZeneca doses produced on license by the SII. The SII was meant to deliver around 560 million doses up to September 2021, constituting the bulk of the Facility's supplies until then. However, this plan was thrown asunder when India was confronted with a resurgence of COVID-19 infections in March, interrupting production and prompting India to restrict vaccine exports.[25] The COVAX Facility was also not able to pivot rapidly to other vaccine manufacturers, as alternatives would cost around "50–100 per cent higher" than the US$3 per dose that the SII charged.[26]

COVAX'S FIRST PHASE: AN "ABYSMAL FAILURE" FOR THE AMC6 IN 1H 2021

The COVAX Facility's stuttering start meant that its actual distribution efforts markedly fell short of its own expectations in 1H, including in Southeast Asia. Four allocation rounds took place over the first six months of 2021. In each allocation round, COVAX would stipulate the type of vaccine and the number of doses that participating countries would be entitled to receive during that cycle.[27] The Pfizer/BioNTech vaccine was allocated in the first and third rounds, while AstraZeneca was the focus of the second and fourth rounds (Table 1).

---

[25] The SII resumed its exports of Covishield to COVAX on 26 November 2021. The almost nine-month-long supply disruption have led some to criticize the Facility's decision to partner the SII as a "mistake". Gavi's Dr Seth Berkley has however defended the "big bet" on AstraZeneca and the SII as "the right thing to do", pointing to the SII's ability to manufacture at scale and the vaccine's developing world-friendly temperature storage profile. See "COVAX Past, Present, and Future".

[26] Olivia Goldhill, "'Naively Ambitious': How COVAX Failed on Its Promise to Vaccinate the World", *STAT*, 8 October 2021, https://www.statnews.com/2021/10/08/how-covax-failed-on-its-promise-to-vaccinate-the-world/

[27] COVAX's internal allocation mechanism involves two bodies, the Joint Allocation Taskforce (JAT) and the Independent Allocation of Vaccine Group (IAVG). The JAT, staffed with personnel from the WHO and Gavi, will prepare the vaccine allocation decision for each round. The IAVG, a panel of twelve external experts, will then review and approve the JAT's proposal.

	Round 1	Round 2	Round 3	Round 4
Duration	Q1 2021	Feb–May 2021	Apr–June 2021	June 2021
Type of Vaccine	Pfizer/ BioNTech	AstraZeneca	Pfizer/ BioNTech	AstraZeneca
No. of Doses Allocated	1,200,420	237,468,000	14,109,030	17,366,400
No. of Recipients	18	142	47	43

Table 2: 1H COVAX Allocations to AMC-Eligible Countries in Southeast Asia

	Round 1	Round 2		Round 3	Round 4	1H Total
	Pfizer/ BioNTech	AstraZeneca-SKBio	SII-Covishield	Pfizer/ BioNTech	AstraZeneca Vaxzevria	
Cambodia			1,104,000		324,000	1,428,000
Indonesia		11,704,800				11,704,800
Laos			480,000	100,620	132,000	712,620
Myanmar		*3,600,000*				*3,600,000*
Philippines	117,000	4,584,000		2,355,210		705,621
Timor-Leste		100,800				100,800
Vietnam		4,176,000				417,600
		AMC6 Total				25,178,430
		AMC6 + Myanmar Total				*28,778,430*

Round 1 was a special round allocating a limited amount of "first-wave" Pfizer/BioNTech doses to eighteen countries early in the year—in the region, only 117,000 Pfizer/BioNTech doses were reserved for the Philippines (Table 2). Meanwhile, Round 3 involved a more comprehensive allocation of 14 million Pfizer/BioNTech shots to forty-seven countries over April to June. Laos and the Philippines were allotted 100,000 and 2.4 million doses, respectively, in the third round.

Round 2 was a regular allocation cycle to distribute 237.5 million doses of AstraZeneca over February to May. All the AMC6 countries (and Myanmar) were promised supplies of the AstraZeneca vaccine, to be produced either by the SII or South Korea's SKBio. Round 4 was scheduled in June as an "exceptional round" to distribute an additional 17 million AstraZeneca doses. This round was meant to address the delayed and/or cancelled shipments of the second round, especially due to the supply disruptions at the SII. Among the AMC6, Laos and Cambodia—the two countries designated to receive SII-Covishield in Round 2—were allocated 24,000 and 132,000 doses, respectively, in Round 4.

The AMC6 countries were collectively promised around 25 million COVAX doses over the four allocation rounds. (If Myanmar is included, the region's total allocation for 1H rises up to 28.8 million doses.) The bulk of the AMC6's 1H entitlement comes from 22.2 million AstraZeneca doses in Round 2. However, the COVAX supply of AstraZeneca during this period was lacklustre and halting, especially for the two AMC6 recipients furnished with the SII-Covishield vaccine.

Both Cambodia and Laos ended up with only slightly more than 20 per cent of their expected AstraZeneca allocation in 1H (Figure 2). Cambodia was promised 1.1 million SII-Covishield shots, but the country—one of the earliest in the world to receive COVAX shots—did not see another shipment in 1H since the delivery of 324,000 doses on 2 March.[28]

---

[28] "Cambodia Among First Countries to Receive COVID-19 Vaccines from COVAX Facility", WHO, 3 March 2021, https://www.who.int/cambodia/news/detail/03-03-2021-cambodia-among-first-countries-to-receive-covid-19-vaccines-from-covax-facility

Figure 2: COVAX Shipments to Cambodia and Laos in 1H 2021

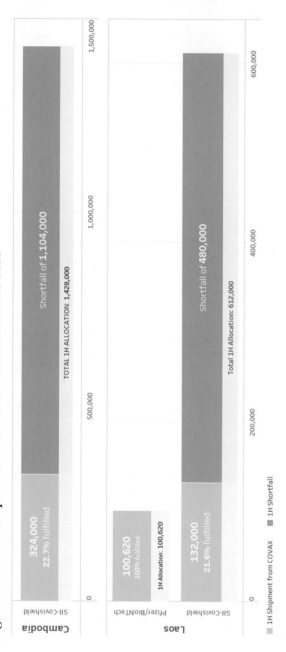

Note: The SII-Covishield allocation figures for Cambodia and Laos are inclusive of their AstraZeneca entitlements that were granted in Round 4.

Laos had a shortfall of 348,000 AstraZeneca shots, obtaining only a single package of 132,000 doses on 20 March.[29] The country was instead provided with 100,620 doses of the mRNA-based Pfizer/BioNTech vaccine on 2 June. For developing countries such as Laos, the ultra-cold chain requirements for mRNA vaccines can impose an unnecessary logistical burden. (In contrast, AstraZeneca can be kept at fridge temperatures.) Additional arrangements were thus needed to be made for Laos to safely receive and deploy the Pfizer/BioNTech shots. The Institut Pasteur du Laos had to reserve two new ultra-cold freezers "specifically for [the Pfizer/BioNTech] vaccines", while the WHO procured an additional three units.[30] The storage requirements also meant that Laos' vaccine rollout would be first limited to Vientiane, the nation's capital, before expanding to "other high-risk areas".

Vietnam, Philippines and Indonesia (whose Round 2 allotments were not dependent on the SII) fared better, receiving between 56 and 70 per cent of their AstraZeneca entitlements (Figure 3). Indonesia received the largest amount of COVAX supplies out of the AMC6, with steady deliveries of between 1 and 4 million shots monthly from March to June. In total, the country received 70 per cent of its entitlement, or around 8.2 million shots out of an expected 11.7 million, in 1H. Be that as it may, this amount was minuscule compared to Indonesia's intention to vaccinate around 208 million residents.

Meanwhile, Vietnam received close to 60 per cent of its allocation, collecting around 2.5 million AstraZeneca doses over two shipments in March and May. For Vietnam, perhaps, the urgency to secure vaccines was not as acute in 1H, owing to Hanoi's successful management of the pandemic up till then. The Philippines similarly secured around

---

[29] "COVID-19 Vaccines Shipped by COVAX Facility Arrive in Lao PDR", UNICEF, 20 March 2021, https://www.unicef.org/laos/press-releases/covid-19-vaccines-shipped-covax-facility-arrive-lao-pdr

[30] "New Shipment of COVID-19 Vaccines from the COVAX Facility Arrive in Lao PDR", UNICEF, 2 June 2021, https://www.unicef.org/laos/press-releases/new-shipment-covid-19-vaccines-covax-facility-arrive-lao-pdr

Figure 3: COVAX Shipments to Indonesia, the Philippines and Vietnam in 1H 2021

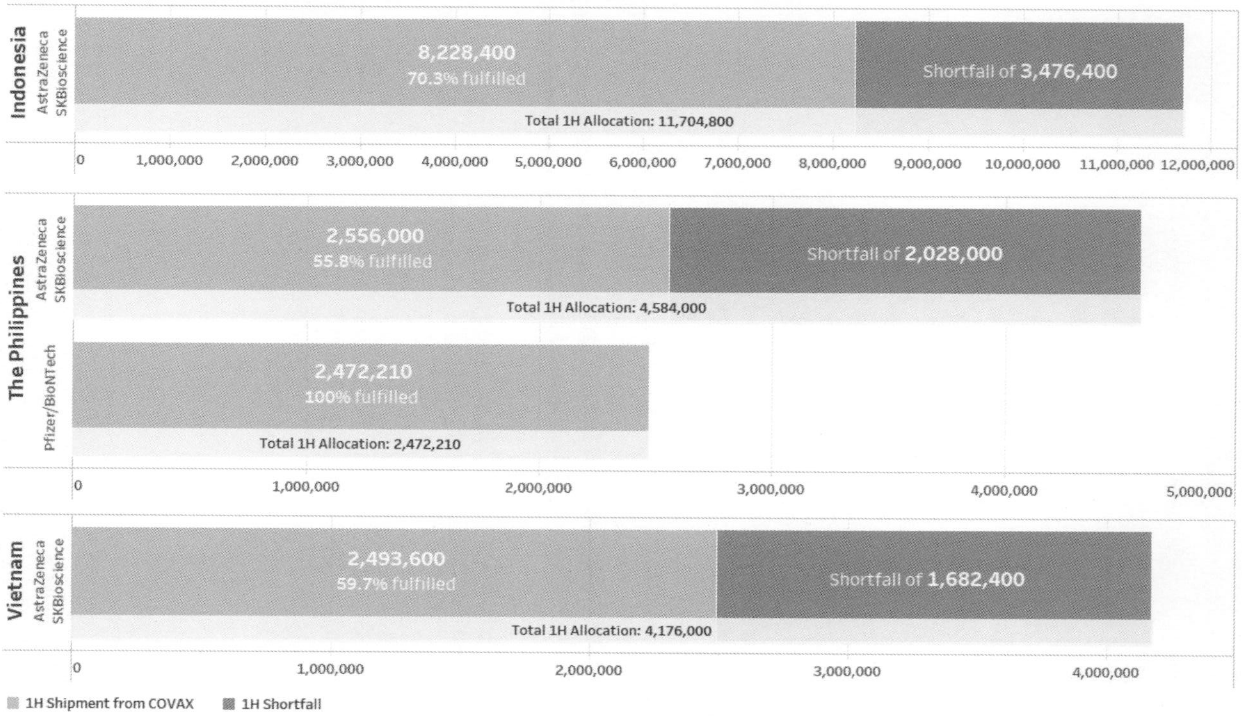

Indonesia
AstraZeneca SKBioscience
8,228,400
70.3% fulfilled
Shortfall of 3,476,400
Total 1H Allocation: 11,704,800
0
1,000,000
2,000,000
3,000,000
4,000,000
5,000,000
6,000,000
7,000,000
8,000,000
9,000,000
10,000,000
11,000,000
12,000,000
The Philippines
AstraZeneca SKBioscience
2,556,000
55.8% fulfilled
Shortfall of 2,028,000
Total 1H Allocation: 4,584,000
Pfizer/BioNTech
2,472,210
100% fulfilled
Total 1H Allocation: 2,472,210
0
1,000,000
2,000,000
3,000,000
4,000,000
5,000,000
Vietnam
AstraZeneca SKBioscience
2,493,600
59.7% fulfilled
Shortfall of 1,682,400
Total 1H Allocation: 4,176,000
0
1,000,000
2,000,000
3,000,000
4,000,000
1H Shipment from COVAX
1H Shortfall

56 per cent of its promised AstraZeneca doses, while receiving its full entitlement of 2.5 million Pfizer/BioNTech shots in May and June.

Timor-Leste was an outlier in the sense that Dili was the only AMC6 recipient provided with supplies exceeding its entitlement (Figure 4). Despite being originally allocated 124,8000 doses, Timor-Leste ended up with 128,000 doses of AstraZeneca in 1H. The excess was made possible by a donation of 24,000 doses from New Zealand on 9 June,[31] in a signal of the Facility's shift to its second phase in the latter half of 2021.

In sum, out of the 25 million COVAX doses allocated to the AMC6 in 1H, the Facility managed to deliver only 16 million—fulfilling only 65.3 per cent of the stipulated entitlement (Figure 5).[32] (The fulfilment figure drops further to 57.1 per cent if Myanmar's entitlement to 3.6 million doses is considered.) As expected, the shortfall was primarily due to the lack of AstraZeneca supplies: the AMC6 were still owed around 8,746,800 AstraZeneca doses as of June.[33]

COVAX'S SECOND PHASE: THE PIVOT TO DOSE DONATIONS

The second phase was primarily driven by wealthier countries releasing their spare vaccine inventories and donating these doses to poorer countries through COVAX. Having recognized its significant supply shortfall by May 2021, the COVAX Facility had shifted its focus towards convincing richer nations to redistribute the excess doses instead of keeping those shots hoarded.

---

[31] "Timor-Leste Receives 100,800 Doses of COVID-19 Vaccines from COVAX, the Largest Single Batch of Vaccine Doses Delivered to the Country to Date", UNICEF, 9 June 2021, https://www.unicef.org/timorleste/press-releases/timor-leste-receives-100800-doses-covid-19-vaccines-covax-largest-single-batch

[32] Annex 1 offers an overview of the schedule and volume of COVAX deliveries to the AMC6 in 1H 2021.

[33] The shortfall increases to 12,346,800 doses if Myanmar's entitlement is included.

Figure 4: COVAX Shipments to Timor-Leste in 1H 2021

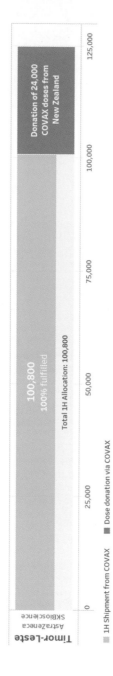
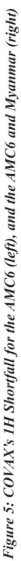

Figure 5: COVAX's 1H Shortfall for the AMC6 (left), and the AMC6 and Myanmar (right)

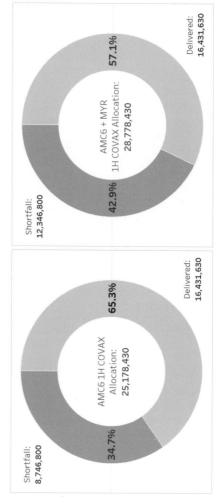

The G7's pledge in June 2021 to donate 1 billion shots, in particular, lent COVAX some renewed momentum.[34] That same month, the United States outlined its commitment to release 80 million shots from its inventory and to facilitate the purchase of 500 million Pfizer/BioNTech shots on the COVAX Facility's behalf for its AMC recipients.[35] In late September, the United States announced that it would be facilitating the procurement of an additional 500 million Pfizer/BioNTech doses, bringing the total sum to 1 billion.[36]

Despite President Biden's pronouncement that these dose donations came with "no strings attached" for recipient countries,[37] they did come with a catch for the COVAX Facility. While the Facility originally had the autonomy to determine how its vaccine supply would be distributed globally, it did not have such discretion with these donated doses. Instead, donors retained the prerogative to "earmark" the specific countries to receive their shots. The United States, for instance, clearly identified that the White House would be the one to "allocate these doses to low and lower-middle income nations around the world, working through COVAX to deliver them".[38]

---

[34] Joseph Lee and Becky Morton, "G7: World Leaders Promise One Billion COVID Vaccine Doses for Poorer Nations", *BBC*, 13 June 2021, https://www.bbc.com/news/uk-57461640

[35] "FACT SHEET: President Biden Announces Historic Vaccine Donation: Half a Billion Pfizer Vaccines to the World's Lowest-Income Nations", The White House, 10 June 2021, https://www.whitehouse.gov/briefing-room/statements-releases/2021/06/10/fact-sheet-president-biden-announces-historic-vaccine-donation-half-a-billion-pfizer-vaccines-to-the-worlds-lowest-income-nations/

[36] Zeke Miller, "Biden Doubles US Global Donation of COVID-19 Vaccine Shots", Associated Press, 23 September 2021, https://apnews.com/article/united-nations-general-assembly-joe-biden-pandemics-business-united-nations-e7c09c1f896d83c0ed80513082787bd3

[37] "Biden Says Pfizer COVID-19 Shots Donated by US Will Ship Globally in August, with 'No Strings Attached'", *Straits Times*, 11 June 2021, https://www.straitstimes.com/world/united-states/biden-says-pfizer-covid-19-shots-donated-by-us-will-ship-globally-in-august-with

[38] "FACT SHEET: President Biden Announces Historic Vaccine Donation".

Still, this pivot to dose donations provided COVAX a lifeline (Figure 6). Of the total 1.5 billion shots that have been allocated by the COVAX Facility in the year up to 15 December,[39] around 56.5 per cent (or 873.6 million) were courtesy of earmarked dose donations.[40] And of the 729 million COVAX shots that had been shipped worldwide by the same date, 58.7 per cent (427 million) were donated.

Earmarked dose donations from the United States alone accounted for 33.8 per cent of all COVAX shipments for the year up to mid-December, followed at a distance by Germany and France in second and third place with 5.7 and 4.1 per cent (Figure 7). The United States' dominant contribution is also reflected in the fact that it was the provider of 57.6 per cent of all dose donations to COVAX (Figure 8).

THE AMC6'S BURGEONING COVAX SUPPLY IN 2H

The Facility's pivot to earmarked dose donations dramatically boosted supplies to the AMC6 in 2H, which collectively received 128 million doses from COVAX in 2H 2021, more than 7.8 times the amount delivered in 1H.[41]

---

[39] Based on its supply forecast, the COVAX Facility tries to allocate doses at least three months in advance to allow recipient countries to prepare for the delivery of the vaccines. There is a time lag between allocation and shipment as recipients need to accept and indicate their readiness to receive the COVAX doses, including agreeing to "the manufacturer-specific indemnity and liability agreement", having the necessary "national regulatory approval for the vaccine", and issuing "an import permit". Only then would COVAX confirm the procurement with the manufacturers and co-ordinate the actual shipment of the doses to recipient countries. See "From Availability to Arrival: How COVAX Doses Make It to Countries", Gavi, https://www.gavi.org/vaccineswork/availability-arrival-how-covax-doses-make-it-countries (accessed 27 December 2021).

[40] The amount of earmarked dose donations reflected here includes those originating from the US-facilitated purchase of the Pfizer/BioNTech vaccine for COVAX.

[41] While the COVAX Facility still conducted allocation rounds in 2H 2021, these are of lesser relevance since most of the AMC6's 2H COVAX supplies came from

Figure 6: Share of Allocated (left) and Shipped (right) COVAX Doses That Were Either from Dose Donations or the COVAX Facility's Own Procurement

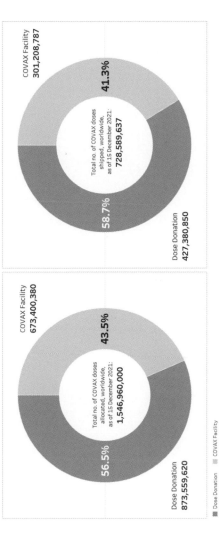

COVAX Facility
673,400,380

43.5%

Total no. of COVAX doses
allocated, worldwide,
as of 15 December 2021:
1,546,960,000

56.5%

Dose Donation
873,559,620

COVAX Facility
301,208,787

41.3%

Total no. of COVAX doses
shipped, worldwide,
as of 15 December 2021:
728,589,637

58.7%

Dose Donation
427,380,850

■ Dose Donation   ■ COVAX Facility

Note: "COVAX Facility" marks the volume of doses that were directly procured by the Facility, while "Dose Donation" indicates those committed by donor countries.

Figure 7: Origins of COVAX Doses Shipped to Recipients (up to 15 December 2021)

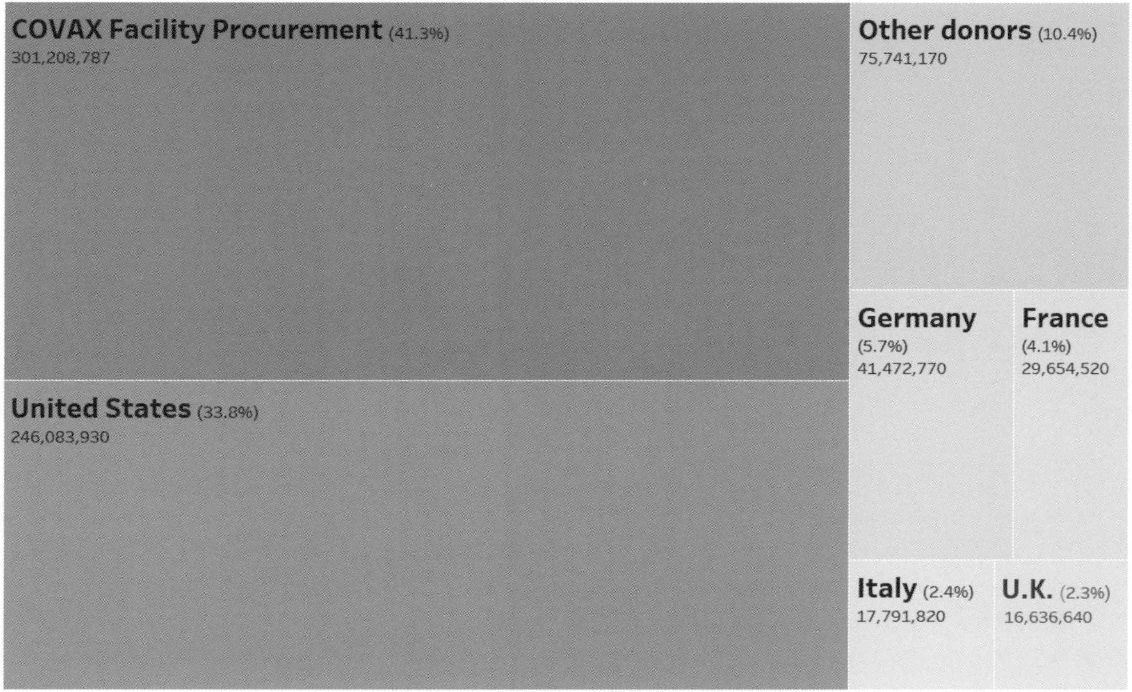

COVAX Facility Procurement (41.3%)
301,208,787

Other donors (10.4%)
75,741,170

Germany
(5.7%)
41,472,770

France
(4.1%)
29,654,520

United States (33.8%)
246,083,930

Italy (2.4%)
17,791,820

U.K. (2.3%)
16,636,640

Figure 8: Individual Donors' Share of COVAX Dose Donations That Were Shipped to Recipients (up to 15 December 2021)

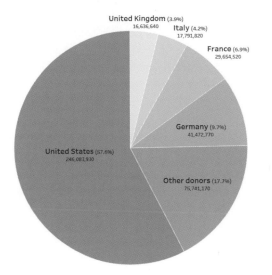

The 2H flow of COVAX shots to the Philippines (45.4 million doses) and Vietnam (36.3 million doses), for instance, were respectively around nine and 14.5 times larger than their 1H supplies (Figure 9). The two countries were the first and third-largest recipients of 2H COVAX doses among the AMC6.[42] Remarkably, 92 per cent of the Philippines'

---

dose donations—which the Facility has no power to allocate due to the practice of earmarking. Hence, measuring the actual volume of COVAX deliveries against the AMC6's expected entitlements in 2H offers limited analytical value. Instead, assessing the share of earmarked dose donations in the AMC6's 2H COVAX provisions would be more useful in understanding the Facility's performance during this period.

[42] Among the AMC6, Indonesia is the second-largest recipient of 2H COVAX doses. However, if corrected for their relative population sizes, the Philippines and Vietnam would occupy the top two spots.

Figure 9: COVAX Shipments to the Philippines and Vietnam in 2H 2021 (up to 15 December)

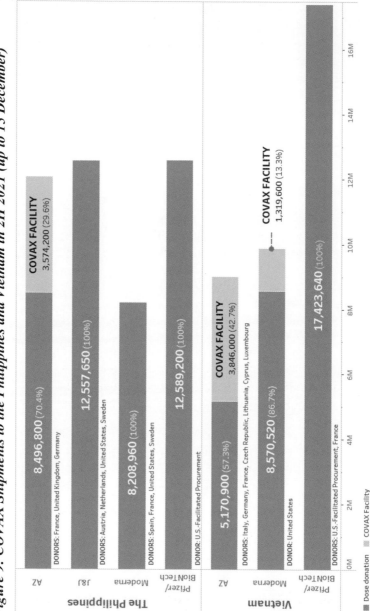

2H COVAX supplies and 85.8 per cent of Vietnam's were supported by earmarked dose donations, testifying presumably to Manila's and Hanoi's strategic salience to the United States and its allies.

Washington alone accounted for 41.4 per cent of the Philippines' 2H COVAX doses, and 61.8 per cent of Vietnam's. The United States provided Manila, a formal treaty ally, with 18.8 million shots of Pfizer/ BioNTech, Moderna and J&J through COVAX. The Biden administration also prioritized Vietnam, dispatching over 16.4 million Pfizer/BioNTech shots through its facilitated purchase with COVAX, and sending 6 out of the 8.5 million Moderna doses that Hanoi received in 2H.

The two countries were also beneficiaries of European largesse, receiving donations from an assortment of countries from the continent. Donated supplies from the United Kingdom, France and Germany of 8.5 million AstraZeneca shots accounted for 70.4 per cent of the Philippines' 2H COVAX inventory of the vaccine. Meanwhile, the septet of Italy, Germany, France, Czech Republic, Lithuania, Cyprus and Luxembourg combined to disburse 5.2 million doses to Vietnam, effectively supplying more than half of the 9 million AstraZeneca shots that Hanoi received in total through COVAX in 2H.

Indonesia received slightly over 40.2 million COVAX doses in 2H (Figure 10). A significant 64.6 per cent of Indonesia's 2H supplies came from dose donations. The generosity of nine European countries and New Zealand provided Indonesia with 7.5 million AstraZeneca shots— accounting for 68.5 per cent of the total 2H COVAX shipment of the vaccine to Jakarta. Among the AstraZeneca donors, France and Italy were the two largest, fronting 3,252,340 and 1,647,500 shots, respectively. Meanwhile, the United States was fully responsible for the archipelago's COVAX provisions of 9.5 million Moderna and 9 million Pfizer/ BioNTech shots. (The latter came from the US-facilitated purchase of the Pfizer/BioNTech vaccine on COVAX's behalf.) Interestingly, Indonesia was the first AMC6 country to be given a Chinese-made vaccine by the Facility, receiving a COVAX shipment of 11 million Sinovac doses in September. These shots were however not dose donations from China, but were instead directly procured by the COVAX Facility.

Cambodia and Laos received around 3 million COVAX shots each in 2H (Figure 11), much lower than the numbers delivered to Indonesia, the

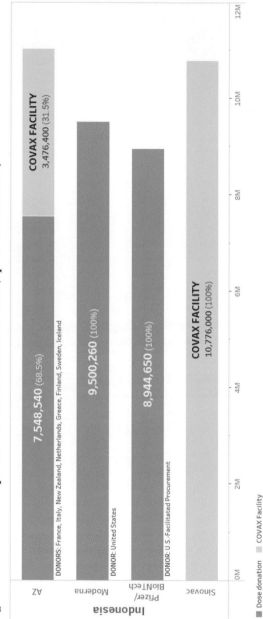

Figure 10: COVAX Shipments to Indonesia in 2H 2021 (up to 15 December)

Figure 11: COVAX Shipments to Cambodia and Laos in 2H 2021 (up to 15 December)

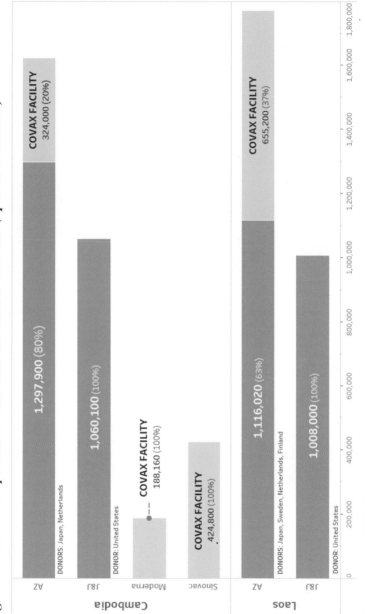

Philippines and Vietnam, but this was still an improvement—especially for Phnom Penh, which saw the delivery of a paltry 324,000 doses in 1H. Out of the 1.6 million AstraZeneca doses Cambodia received from COVAX in 2H, 80 per cent were donated by Japan and the Netherlands. The United States also donated the entirety of Phnom Penh's COVAX stock of 1 million-odd J&J doses. In total, 71.6 per cent of Cambodia's 2H COVAX supply were donated. (Cambodia was also the second AMC6 country after Indonesia to receive Facility-procured Sinovac shots.)

Earmarked donations similarly occupied a 76.4 per cent share of Laos' 2H COVAX supply. Finland, Japan, the Netherlands, and Spain collectively donated 63 per cent of the 1.8 million AstraZeneca doses that Vientiane received, while the United States sent the land-locked country 1 million J&J shots through COVAX.

For Timor-Leste, all of its 2H COVAX doses were supplied through earmarked donations (Figure 12). The tiny country of 1.3 million received a shipment of 168,000 AstraZeneca doses from Japan in August, and 100,620 Pfizer shots from the United States in October (with an additional 100,000 Pfizer doses expected to arrive in Dili in the future).

In aggregate,[43] COVAX shipments to the AMC6 totalled 128 million doses in 2H, with almost 104 million—a staggering 80.8 per cent— coming from dose donations (Figure 13). Given the dismal 1H delivery of 16.4 million COVAX shots, the trend holds true even if we were to consider the figures from the 1H and 2H periods together: for the year up to 15 December,[44] the AMC6 received around 145 million COVAX doses, of which 104 million (71.7 per cent) were donated. That was enough to provide first dose coverage for 28.6 per cent of the total population of the AMC6.

---

[43] Annex 2 offers an overview of the schedule and volume of COVAX deliveries to the AMC6 in 2H 2021. Annex 3 lists out the origins and the volumes of earmarked dose donations to the AMC6.

[44] It is quite likely that when 2021 is considered in full, the proportion of donated doses would increase given that the projections at the time of writing indicate that some AMC6 countries are due for further shipments of earmarked COVAX dose donations in the second half of December.

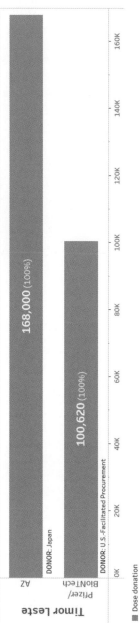

Figure 12: COVAX Shipments to Timor-Leste in 2H 2021 (up to 15 December)

Figure 13: The Origins of COVAX Shipments to Individual AMC6 Countries in 2H, and in the Aggregate for the Year (up to 15 December)

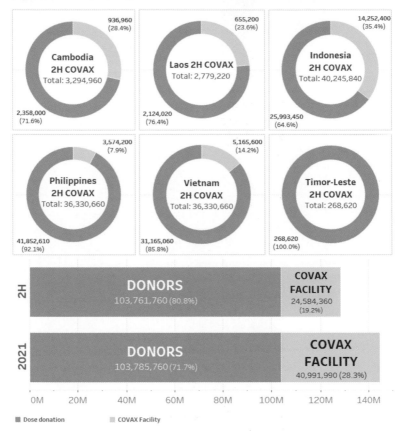

The United States powered the flow of donated COVAX doses to the AMC6: its roughly 62 million shots constituted almost 60 per cent of all the donated shots shipped to the region in 2021 (Figure 14) Germany, the Netherlands and France each contributed around 8 per cent to the AMC6's donated COVAX supplies, while the United Kingdom accounted for 5 per cent with its donation of 5 million-odd AstraZeneca shots to the Philippines.

Figure 14: Major COVAX Dose Donors to the AMC6

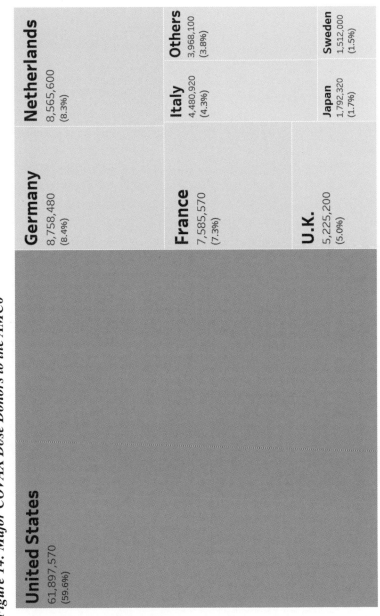

Germany 8,758,480 (8.4%)	**Netherlands** 8,565,600 (8.3%)	
France 7,585,570 (7.3%)	**Italy** 4,480,920 (4.3%)	**Others** 3,968,100 (3.8%)
U.K. 5,225,200 (5.0%)	**Japan** 1,792,320 (1.7%)	**Sweden** 1,512,000 (1.5%)
United States 61,897,570 (59.6%)		

Collectively, the AMC6 accounted for 24.3 per cent of all dose donations delivered worldwide through COVAX in 2021. The fact that these six countries, despite making up only 7 per cent of the world's population, were earmarked for 25 per cent of the COVAX shots donated by the United States lends confirmation that COVAX 2.0—a donation-driven model in which donors can earmark their doses to their preferred recipients—had presented the region with a prodigious boon.

W(H)ITHER COVAX 2.0?

The AMC6 have benefitted tremendously from the second phase pivot to dose donations, but it is important to recognize that this shift, and the transformation to COVAX 2.0 more generally, has complicated the Facility's operations and its future prospects. Though Seth Berkley of Gavi has described the turn to donations as an "interim" measure before the Facility's own "advance-purchase agreements ... came through",[45] the figures reveal that COVAX is still overwhelmingly reliant on earmarked dose supplies from Western countries.

For one, the earmarking of dose donations—as advantageous as it has been for the AMC6—has caused considerable planning and logistical difficulties for the Facility. Because donors release their excess doses through COVAX outside the ambit of the Facility's formal allocation processes, COVAX officials have to constantly revise their distribution plans to account for the flow of earmarked doses. Seth Berkley has mentioned, perhaps only half-in-jest, that COVAX's "forecasts are changing on a daily basis—sometimes on an hourly basis".[46] Moreover, due to its lack of oversight and control over these donations, the Facility has to occasionally scramble to help recipient countries deploy these donated shots before they expire—as was the case for some African countries which received dose shipments from the United Kingdom and Canada that only had weeks remaining in their shelf-life. Some

---

[45] "COVAX Past, Present, and Future".

[46] Ibid.

donors also do not cover the freight and transportation expenses of their donations, saddling the already-overstretched Facility with additional "fringe costs".[47] More recently, two African health organizations joined the COVAX Facility in complaining that the dose donations to the continent have been "ad hoc, provided with little notice and short shelf lives", and often offered without the "essential ancillaries" such as syringes and diluent.[48]

These concerns are not unknown to the donors. The Facility's Independent Allocation of Vaccines Group (IAVG), the panel of experts which provides approval to all of COVAX's internal allocation decisions, issued a public reminder on 24 September that the dose donations "should complement rather than replace vaccine procurement by COVAX", while tersely grousing about "the high transaction burden and costs in managing these donations".[49] The IAVG also beseeched donors "to reduce/remove all earmarking" and ensure that the bequeathed doses have an "adequate shelf life", but has met with little success.

---

[47] Goldhill, "Naively Ambitious".

[48] "Joint Statement on Dose Donations of COVID-19 Vaccines to African Countries", WHO, 29 November 2021, https://www.who.int/news/item/29-11-2021-joint-statement-on-dose-donations-of-covid-19-vaccines-to-african-countries

[49] "What Needs to Change to Enhance COVID-19 Vaccine Access", WHO, 24 September 2021, https://www.who.int/news/item/24-09-2021-what-needs-to-change-to-enhance-covid-19-vaccine-access. The IAVG also emphasized the need developing countries have to access the necessary funding and technical support to actually deploy the doses that they are receiving. The IAVG has been expressing these concerns since July, after dose donations began flowing. See "Report of the Independent Allocation of Vaccines Group on the Allocation of COVAX Facility Secured Vaccines", WHO, 15 July 2021, https://www.who.int/publications/m/item/report-of-the-independent-allocation-of-vaccines-group-on-the-allocation-of-covax-facility-secured-vaccines-15-july-2021; and 29 July 2021, https://www.who.int/publications/m/item/report-of-the-independent-allocation-of-vaccines-group-on-the-allocation-of-covax-facility-secured-vaccines-29-july-2021

More importantly, earmarked dose donations severely undermine the Facility's institutional autonomy. It should be recalled that COVAX was initially mooted as an instrument of global solidarity, operating as a genuine vaccine hub for the world in which doses would be shared equitably, and no country would receive special priority.[50] However, because COVAX 2.0 "has had to rely on the variable goodwill of its wealthiest partners", this has effectively transformed COVAX from a solidarity mechanism into an "an *aid* project" (emphasis original),[51] leaving the countries of the Global South at the grace of the Global North—or more accurately, the latter's determination of the former's geostrategic worth.

There are also other donor decisions that have supercharged COVAX supplies, but at the expense of its autonomy. For instance, the first US-facilitated procurement of 500 million Pfizer/BioNTech doses for COVAX in June measurably bolstered the Facility's progress to meet its milestone of delivering 2 billion doses. However, to finance this purchase, the United States diverted around half of its US$4 billion pledge to the AMC—so not only did Washington remove from the COVAX Facility the discretion to determine how these Pfizer/BioNTech shots are distributed, but it also scuppered the Facility's financial ability to procure vaccines independently.[52] Similarly, it was revealed that

---

[50] See, for instance, "Fair Allocation Mechanism for COVID-19 Vaccines through the COVAX", WHO, 9 September 2020, https://www.who.int/publications/m/item/fair-allocation-mechanism-for-covid-19-vaccines-through-the-covax-facility; and "Allocation Logic and Algorithm to Support Allocation of Vaccines Secured through the COVAX Facility", WHO, 15 February 2021, https://www.who.int/publications/m/item/allocation-logic-and-algorithm-to-support-allocation-of-vaccines-secured-through-the-covax-facility. More details about COVAX's allocation mechanisms, policies and principles can be found at https://www.who.int/groups/iavg

[51] Storeng, Puyvallée and Stein, "COVAX and the Rise of the 'Super Public Private Partnership'", pp. 7, 8.

[52] See "Biden Says Pfizer COVID-19 Shots Donated by US Will Ship Globally in August". In general, public details about the specific arrangements of the US Government's facilitated purchase of Pfizer/BioNTech for COVAX are

the United States' second facilitated procurement in September also involved the funding diversion of "hundreds of millions of dollars" that were previously pledged to beefing up the vaccination infrastructure in developing countries.[53]

As the Facility's autonomy diminishes, there is a profound risk that COVAX will be reduced to (or at least be seen as) a mere logistical apparatus for the United States and its partners to route their selective vaccine donations. This perception that COVAX is functioning as the fulfilment arm of the West's vaccine diplomacy has been strengthened by the unfortunate insistence of some countries for "branding visibility" on their donations, such as stamping their national emblems on the deliveries.[54]

It has not been lost on some that the current arrangements have largely consigned COVAX into the role of a logistical intermediary, and one that is potentially superfluous. For instance, Tokyo has displayed scant interest in channelling its excess doses through COVAX. It has chosen to donate 11 million AstraZeneca doses directly to Indonesia, Vietnam and the Philippines, while committing only 1.8 million doses

---

scarce. The IAVG Report for Allocation Round 5 explicitly indicated that all the facilitated doses allocated in that cycle were "earmarked by the USG [US Government] to AMC participants as well as six self-financing participants (SFPs) in the African Union". In subsequent rounds involving more of these facilitated doses, it is not clear whether the United States continued to exercise its earmarking prerogatives, although the IAVG alluded to the "limitations of the Pfizer USG's supply earmarking" in their Round 10 report. Requests for clarification from COVAX, as well as some regional WHO and UNICEF officials, have not been successful.

[53] Benjamin Mueller and Rebecca Robbins, "Where a Vast Global Vaccination Program Went Wrong", *New York Times*, 2 August 2021, https://www.nytimes.com/2021/08/02/world/europe/covax-covid-vaccine-problems-africa.html. The report also explained how the United States became involved in the facilitated procurement, after "tension" emerged between Pfizer/BioNTech and COVAX.

[54] Storeng, Puyvallée and Stein, "COVAX and the Rise of the 'Super Public Private Partnership'", p. 9.

Figure 15: Japan's Bilateral (in Lighter Grey) and COVAX-Routed Dose Donations (in Darker Grey) to the AMC6 (up to 15 December)

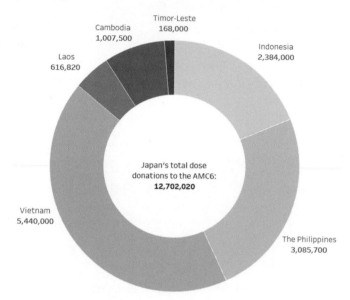

Timor-Leste 168,000
Cambodia 1,007,500
Laos 616,820
Indonesia 2,384,000

Japan's total dose donations to the AMC6: 12,702,020

Vietnam 5,440,000

The Philippines 3,085,700

through COVAX for Cambodia, Laos and Timor-Leste (Figure 15). In perhaps another indication of its indifference to COVAX, Tokyo's (as yet unfulfilled) promise to donate 10,000 doses through the Facility to Vietnam stands in pale comparison to the 5.4 million doses to Vietnam that it has already dispatched directly to Hanoi. The Japanese foreign minister had justified the country's preference for bilateral donations in June with the rationale that if Tokyo were to "go through an international organization, the procedures in getting approval may take time".[55] This

---

[55] "Japan to Ship 1 mln COVID-19 Vaccines to Vietnam on Wednesday", Reuters, 15 June 2021, https://www.reuters.com/world/asia-pacific/japan-ship-1-mln-covid-19-vaccines-vietnam-june-16-2021-06-15/

justification is provided even though, strictly speaking, there is no requisite for an "approval"—the Facility lacks the ability or even the authority to give such approvals.

COVAX 2.0: A BOON WITH HIDDEN COSTS AND CONSEQUENCES?

The pivot to earmarked dose donations released much-needed vaccines to the developing world, and precipitated an outsized flow of shots into Southeast Asian countries in particular. However, the reliance on dose donations and the practice of earmarking has prevented COVAX from living up to its aspiration of fostering vaccine equity. The diversion away from the principle of equity is one of the significant hidden costs of COVAX 2.0.

The AMC6, as benefactors, lack the capacity to determine or re-orientate COVAX's strategic trajectory. Neither are they (or any other developing country) in a position to reject these dose donations in the name of global vaccine equity. And they should not—no country can be expected to sacrifice its urgent national needs for enlightened imperatives such as the multilaterally coordinated equitable provision of global public goods. Nevertheless, it remains important to acknowledge that the evolution to COVAX 2.0 carries its own future risks and consequences, especially since these potential outcomes may blunt the immediate advantages that the new COVAX regime is proffering.

Southeast Asia has prudential reason to take the cause of vaccine equity seriously. Firstly, more than being just a moral imperative, vaccine equity is a "practical necessity" since inequitable access to vaccines "is not merely unjust but hazardous".[56] Large pools of the unvaccinated across the world offer a ready bio-reservoir for the coronavirus to constantly evolve and mutate, risking the emergence of newer variants

---

[56] Michael T. Osterholm and Mark Olshaker, "The Pandemic That Won't End", *Foreign Affairs*, 8 March 2021, https://www.foreignaffairs.com/articles/world/2021-03-08/pandemic-wont-end

that could be more transmissible or virulent—or worse, resistant to existing vaccines. Given the hyper-mobility of people and products in a globalized world, no outbreak can be contained within or kept outside national boundaries; global recovery requires global vaccine access. "No one is safe until everyone is safe" may sound like a tired refrain, but its truth has been demonstrated by how the emergence and proliferation of the Delta and Delta Plus variants have prolonged the pandemic—a scenario likely to recur with Omicron.

Secondly, the principle of vaccine equity can help preserve the region's interests in future pandemic outbreaks, especially given the WHO's December 2020 warning that COVID-19 is "not necessarily the big one".[57] The AMC6's COVAX donation windfall is more a function of geopolitical courtship by the United States as it seeks to rebuff Chinese influence in the region. However, it is not at all certain that the region will endure as a contested space; likewise, neither can it be said with confidence that Southeast Asia will find favour with competing major powers in the future, or command a similar amount of their attention and interest.

Thirdly, on a related note, fortifying the independence and neutrality of a multilateral institution such as COVAX and investing it with the authority to co-ordinate support and supplies in crises enhances the region's strategic autonomy. Having an assured reliable source of vaccines (and more generally, medical equipment and tools) means that the region's public health will not be held hostage by the strategic whims of external powers or has to rely on largesse arising from contests of vaccine (or other forms of medical) diplomacy.

An institutionally strengthened COVAX can also benefit the region by addressing certain underlying issues that have contributed to the vaccine supply constraints, thus creating an improved global vaccine regime that

---

[57] Melissa Davey, "WHO Warns COVID-19 Pandemic Is 'Not Necessarily the Big One'", *Guardian*, 29 December 2020, https://www.theguardian.com/world/2020/dec/29/who-warns-covid-19-pandemic-is-not-necessarily-the-big-one

is more "fit for purpose".[58] For instance, a consolidated COVAX may be able to push for and co-ordinate the diversification of the vaccine manufacturing base beyond the current "producers' club" of thirteen territories.[59] None of the thirteen is located in Southeast Asia. Gavi's Seth Berkley has mused about "regional manufacturing" as a possibility to relieve production pressures in the future.[60] This could nicely dovetail with regional countries' efforts to assume more responsibilities for vaccine production locally. Indonesia and Malaysia have, for example, established fill-and-finish arrangements with China for the Sinovac vaccine, with Jakarta recently professing ambitions to become a "global vaccine [production] hub" for the WHO.[61] Meanwhile, Singapore's new BioNTech installation will start churning out COVID-19 vaccines in 2023; this is also a possibility for Vietnam, as the country's largest conglomerate Vingroup has partnered US-based Arcturus Therapeutics to manufacture Arcturus' mRNA vaccine candidate.[62] A more collectivized approach to vaccine production and knowledge-sharing may help to avoid

---

[58] Osterholm and Olshaker, "The Pandemic That Won't End".

[59] Simon J. Evenett, Bernard Hoekman, Nadia Rocha, and Michele Ruta, "The COVID-19 Vaccine Production Club: Will Value Chains Temper Nationalism?", European University Institute Working Paper RSC 2021/36, March 2021, https://cadmus.eui.eu/handle/1814/70363. The thirteen are Argentina, Australia, Brazil, Canada, China, the European Union, India, Japan, Korea, the Russian Federation, the United Kingdom and the United States.

[60] "COVAX Past, Present, and Future".

[61] Tom Allard and Kate Lamb, "Indonesia in Talks with WHO to Become Global Vaccine Hub: Minister", Reuters, 16 September 2021, https://www.reuters.com/world/asia-pacific/exclusive-indonesia-talks-with-who-become-global-vaccine-hub-minister-2021-09-16/

[62] "Written Reply to PQ on Vaccine Manufacturing Capabilities", Minister of Trade and Industry (Singapore), 5 October 2021, https://www.mti.gov.sg/Newsroom/Parliamentary-Replies/2021/10/Oral-reply-to-PQ-on-vaccine-manufacturing-capabilities; Giang Nguyen, "Arcturus Allows Vietnam's Vingroup to Make COVID Vaccines", *Bloomberg*, 2 August 2021, https://www.bloomberg.com/news/articles/2021-08-02/arcturus-agrees-to-let-vietnam-s-vingroup-produce-its-vaccines

misadventures such as the one at Siam BioScience, which struggled early in the year to produce the AstraZeneca vaccine on license.[63] Relatedly, if COVAX does mature into a genuine global node for vaccine distribution, its enhanced purchasing scale can temper corporate interests towards the direction of serving the developing world, for example through patent waivers and technology transfers.

To be fair, the COVAX Facility has been and will always be constrained by the fact that it is a multilateral institution with no inherently endowed resources or enforcement authority to compel powerful nations to act for the global good. On the contrary, it relies primarily on the goodwill and magnanimity of these same countries to undertake its work properly. COVAX is thus not impervious to the interests and agendas of the major powers. Multilateral governance is a difficult act to pull off even at the best of times when interests converge, and good intentions on the Facility's part alone are not enough to prevail over geopolitical realities and the imperfect conditions in which multilateral undertakings are exercised.

The challenge of building COVAX up from scratch during a pandemic has been compared to "building a sailboat when you're in a storm in the middle of the high seas".[64] The COVAX Facility has had to be adaptable and nimble to ensure that the vaccines are indeed reaching the developing world. The pivot to dose donations was a necessary improvisation to improve the chances that more residents of the Global South could get a shot, even if the flow of earmarked supplies could be characterized as inequitable. (After all, this is better than having an equitable lack of vaccines.)

With the growing need for booster shots likely to arise in the coming months, COVAX and the developed world face a stern test. Will richer

---

[63] John Reed, Michael Peel, and Hannah Kuchler, "A King's Vaccine: Thailand's Struggle to Deliver Jabs to Its People", *Financial Times*, 10 June 2021, https://www.ft.com/content/aaa8b820-68c7-408d-9486-222fe2d65634

[64] "COVAX Past, Present, and Future".

nations return to the early days of vaccine hoarding, or is COVAX capable of securing sufficient supplies to relieve the needs of the developing world? This would be a valuable opportunity for fixing the COVAX sail mast and repair its rudders and propellers, so that it can be in better stead for future public health crises.

Annex 1: Raw Data of COVAX Deliveries to the AMC6 and Myanmar in 1H 2021

		Mar 21	Apr 21	May 21	Jun 21	Delivery 1H	Allocation 1H	Shortfall	Fulfilled
Cambodia	SII-Covishield	324,000	–	–	–	324,000	1,428,000	1,104,000	22.7%
Indonesia	AstraZeneca	1,113,600	3,852,000	1,444,900	1,817,900	8,228,400	11,704,800	3,476,400	70.3%
Laos	SII-Covishield	132,000	–	–	–	132,000	612,000	480,000	21.6%
	Pfizer/BioNTech	–	–	100,620	–	100,620	100,620	0	100%
Myanmar	SII-Covishield	–	–	–	–	0	3,600,000	3,600,000	0%
The Philippines	AstraZeneca	525,600	–	2,030,400	–	2,556,000	4,584,000	2,028,000	55.8%
	Pfizer/BioNTech	–	–	193,050	2,279,160	2,472,210	2,472,210	0	100%
Timor-Leste	AstraZeneca	–	24,000	–	100,800	124,800	100,800	-24,000	123.8%
Vietnam	AstraZeneca	811,200	–	1,682,400	–	2,493,600	4,176,000	1,682,400	59.7%
AMC6 + Myanmar Total						16,431,630	28,778,430	12,346,800	57.1%
AMC 6 Total (without Myanmar)							25,178,430	8,746,800	65.3%

Annex 2: Raw Data of COVAX Deliveries to the AMC6 in 2H 2021

		Jul 21	Aug 21	Sep 21	Oct 21	Nov 21	Dec 21	2H Total	Donated	%
CAM	AstraZeneca Vaxzevria	332,000	675,500			324,000	290,400	1,621,900	1,297,900	80%
	Janssen (J&J)	450,500	609,600					1,060,100	1,060,100	100%
	Sinovac				124,800		300,000	424,800		
	Moderna					188,160		188,160		
IND	AstraZeneca Vaxzevria	3,476,400		3,360,340	1,373,200	1,065,400	1,749,600	11,024,940	7,548,540	68.5%
	Moderna	4,500,160	3,500,000				1,500,100	9,500,260	9,500,260	100%
	Pfizer/BioNTech			4,644,900	800,280	3,499,470		8,944,650	8,944,650	100%
	Sinovac			10,776,000				10,776,000		
LAO	AstraZeneca Vaxzevria		616,820		523,200	631,200		1,771,220	1,116,020	63%
	Janssen (J&J)	1,008,000						1,008,000	1,008,000	100 %
PHP	AstraZeneca Vaxzevria	2,028,000			2,391,000	6,019,100	1,632,900	12,071,000	8,496,800	70.4%
	Pfizer/BioNTech			2,770,560	9,516,780	301,860		12,589,200	12,589,200	100%
	Moderna		3,000,060				5,208,900	8,208,960	8,208,960	100%
	Janssen (J&J)	3,240,850					9,316,800	12,557,650	12,557,650	100%
TL	AstraZeneca Vaxzevria		168,000					168,000	168,000	100%
	Pfizer/BioNTech				100,620			100,620	100,620	100%
VTN	AstraZeneca Vaxzevria		1,682,400	2,366,540	4,154,960		813,000	9,016,900	5,170,900	57.3%
	Moderna	5,000,100				2,319,620	2,570,400	9,890,120	8,570,520	86.7%
	Pfizer/BioNTech		1,065,870		6,133,140	7,993,440	2,231,190	17,423,640	17,423,640	100%
	AMC6 Total							128,346,120	103,761,760	80.9%

Annex 3: Raw Data of COVAX Dose Donations to the AMC6 Which Have Been Delivered

Donor	Recipient	Vaccine	No. of Doses Donated Via COVAX	Total
Austria	Philippines	J&J	266,400	266,400
Cyprus	Vietnam	AstraZeneca	85,300	85,300
Czechia	Vietnam	AstraZeneca	460,800	460,800
Finland	Indonesia	AstraZeneca	259,200	360,000
	Laos	AstraZeneca	100,800	
France	Indonesia	AstraZeneca	3,252,340	7,585,570
	Philippines	Moderna	1,058,400	
	Philippines	AstraZeneca	1,632,900	
	Vietnam	AstraZeneca	672,000	
	Vietnam	Pfizer/BioNTech	969,930	
Germany	Philippines	AstraZeneca	1,638,700	8,758,480
	Philippines	Moderna	3,696,900	
	Vietnam	AstraZeneca	852,480	
	Vietnam	Moderna	2,570,400	
Greece	Indonesia	AstraZeneca	444,000	444,000
Iceland	Indonesia	AstraZeneca	14,400	127,200
	Indonesia	AstraZeneca	112,800	
Italy	Indonesia	AstraZeneca	1,647,500	4,480,920
	Vietnam	AstraZeneca	2,833,420	
Japan	Cambodia	AstraZeneca	1,007,500	1,792,320
	Laos	AstraZeneca	616,820	
	Timor-Leste	AstraZeneca	168,000	
Lithuania	Vietnam	AstraZeneca	235,700	235,700
Luxembourg	Vietnam	AstraZeneca	31,200	31,200

Netherlands	Cambodia	AstraZeneca	290,400	8,565,600
	Indonesia	AstraZeneca	537,600	
	Laos	AstraZeneca	199,200	
	Philippines	J&J	7,538,400	
New Zealand	Indonesia	AstraZeneca	684,400	708,400
	Timor-Leste	AstraZeneca	24,000	
Spain	Philippines	Moderna	453,600	453,600
Sweden	Indonesia	AstraZeneca	214,700	413,900
	Laos	AstraZeneca	199,200	
Sweden	Philippines	J&J	1,512,000	1,512,000
Switzerland	Indonesia	AstraZeneca	381,600	381,600
United Kingdom	Philippines	AstraZeneca	5,225,200	5,225,200
United States of America	Cambodia	J&J	1,060,100	61,897,570
	Indonesia	Moderna	9,500,260	
	Indonesia	Pfizer/BioNTech	8,944,650	
	Laos	J&J	1,008,000	
	Philippines	Pfizer/BioNTech	12,589,200	
	Philippines	J&J	3,240,850	
	Philippines	Moderna	3,000,060	
	Timor-Leste	Pfizer/BioNTech	100,620	
	Vietnam	Pfizer/BioNTech	16,453,710	
	Vietnam	Moderna	6,000,120